Men's Health over 50
Stay Healthy and Fit For Life

by CW Piper

Contents

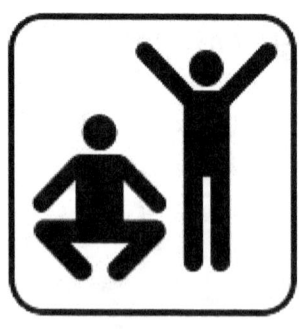

Introduction

The good news is that you have made it this far, so congratulations!

However, as it is only natural that more health problems will occur as you become older, you may be wondering how best to maintain good health at and beyond the age of 50.

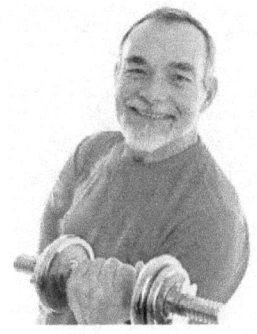

Good health is a natural consequence of a healthy lifestyle, which involves of course healthy eating and regular exercise. It takes a bit more effort and discipline to stay healthy when you are over 50, but the rewards that you get in return are well worth the extra effort.

When I joined this exclusive club a few years ago now, I got to thinking, and always find the best way for me to absorb information is by writing it down - or in other words, researching and writing a book!

In this book there are 3 main areas I will cover:

First up is advice about eating - you should naturally always try to include a variety of vegetables, fruits, whole grains, and low-fat meat and dairy products (where appropriate). Eat just enough food to satisfy. Eating the right food and getting rid of bad habits can help you overcome a lot of potential health problems, but you still need to lead an active lifestyle to achieve optimal health.

So the second part of this book is about appropriate exercise - aim for at least some moderate-intensity physical activity, such as walking, every day of the week.

Regular exercise can improve your blood circulation, stimulate metabolism, improve tone and strengthen your muscles, and also burn excess calories.

It is recommended that you do 30 minutes to 1 hour of 'cardiovascular' exercises every day.

Then I briefly discuss weight balance as a separate topic, and reference the concerns we have as men over 50, and what to do about them, if anything.

Finally, and equally important in my opinion, you should engage in some mentally stimulating activities on a daily basis to keep your mind sharp and healthy, whether it is reading, playing with mind puzzles or studying something interesting and new.

In the Appendices I pass on some useful tips on walking and stretching to help get you started today.

Enjoy and do check out my website for more info.

CW.

Chapter 1 – Eating Well

It all starts with a healthy diet - without food we would cease to function, and eating the right types and quantities of food is a critical part of getting and staying healthy. Following a healthy diet is then a very important part of maintaining good health.

When you are over 50 years old, the metabolism of your body will not be the same as when you were in your 30s or 40s. As such, your body will need different nutrients to stay healthy, and you have to eat certain types of food to ensure that all your nutritional needs will be met.

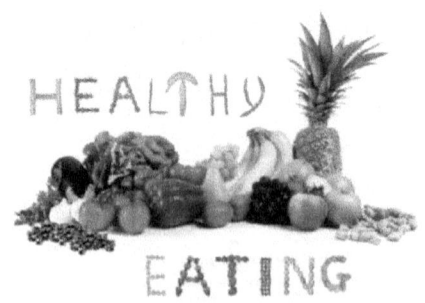

You certainly should try to consume all of the right foods such as vegetables, fruits, whole grains, and low-fat meat and dairy products where appropriate. Eating the right food and maybe finally shedding some of those bad habits will help you to avoid a lot of potential health problems, and you still need to lead an active lifestyle to achieve optimal health.

In the Appendices I give some tips on beginning an easy exercise routine such as walking and stretching to get you started being healthier from today.

I refer to it as food to enjoy because this is what your approach needs to be – if you don't learn to enjoy your food regime, then you won't last long with it – so this is my key message for you to take away.

Learn to enjoy the food you choose to eat.

1.2 Plants

Vegetables

There are so many great and wonderful vegetables you can buy in your local store these days, and you should enjoy this huge variety to the full, I am not going to list them all here.

Some veggies that you should definitely include in your daily diet are the dark green ones - like spinach, kale, broccoli, cabbage and beans.

Even if you do not like a particular vegetable, always try to rediscover some of those that you may have avoided in your life until now, you may even realise that you start to like them.

I did not like being force fed green vegetables by my own parents, and in retaliation I believed that I did not like them (broccoli and spinach come to mind).

However once I made my own way in the world I soon discovered that I really did enjoy food (helped that I knew that it was good for me), and in fact even started growing those dark greens in my own garden. I also discovered garlic after childhood, but that is a whole book on its own!

Fruit

Of the many fruits easily available today, ones that you should regularly consume include oranges, apples, grapes, watermelon, peaches, berries (all kinds) and pears.

There is a belief nowadays that citrus fruit is not great for arthritis, but as long as it is not the first food you eat or drink in the morning, the benefits of citrus in your body will outweigh any of these concerns.

It is also important that you eat more whole grain foods, such as brown rice, oatmeal and whole wheat. Whole grains are known to have very low fat content, and they contain good amounts of fibre, protein, vitamins and minerals that can benefit your health in many ways.

All the latest evidence suggests that a plant-based diet, rich in fruits, vegetables, whole grains, and plant oils, will help to reduce the risk of male health concerns, including heart disease, stroke, diabetes, and cancer. So adding fresh fruits and vegetables is a no-brainer for adopting a plant-based diet, but don't neglect nuts, seeds, and legumes.

Nuts and Seeds

It doesn't pay to obsess over exact portions of nuts and seeds to eat. Sprinkle a loose handful of nuts on your morning cereal, yogurt, or oatmeal, as is a tablespoon of sunflower or chia seeds.

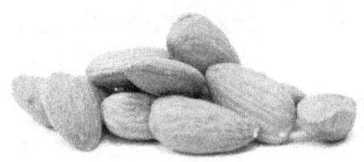

Nuts are full of goodness, and while they can be fattening taken in careful amounts, nuts can be an essential part of a healthy weight-loss program. They are high in calories and fat, but most nuts contain healthy fats that do not clog arteries.

Nuts are also good sources of protein, dietary fibre and minerals, including magnesium and copper. One-half ounce of mixed nuts has about 84 calories.

Seeds may be tiny but they are real nutritional powerhouses - loaded with healthy fats, fiber, protein and minerals. Use for snacking or sprinkle them into your dishes.

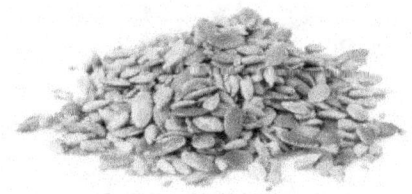

I am not going to go into great detail, but consider trying out sunflower seeds, chia or pumpkin seeds and use on a regular basis, if not every day.

1.3 Meat

<u>Eating Meat:</u>

If, like me, you do enjoy meat, maybe try to limit your meat exposure somewhat, and avoid eating meat all the time.

As you get older and if you are a meat eater - you should also endeavour wherever it is possible to eat lean meats, such as chicken and turkey, and fresh fish, because they contain less fat and cholesterol. Choose cuts of meat that are lower in fat and trim off all the visible fat. Lower fat meats include pork tenderloin and beef round steak, sirloin, flank steak, and extra lean ground beef. Also, pay attention to portion sizes.

Also it is strongly advisable that you use heart-friendly natural oils, such as olive oil, to do your cooking.

Eating red meat generally makes it harder to lose weight. Eating lean meat in small amounts can be part of a healthy weight-loss plan. Red meat, pork, chicken, and fish contain some cholesterol and saturated fat (the least healthy kind of fat). They also contain healthy nutrients like protein, iron, and zinc.

Not Eating Meat:

Vegetarians - like non-vegetarians - can also make food choices that contribute to weight gain, like eating large amounts of high-fat, high-calorie foods or foods with little or no nutritional value.

Vegetarian diets should be as carefully planned as non-vegetarian diets to make sure they are balanced. Nutrients that non-vegetarians normally get from animal products, but that are not always found in a vegetarian eating plan, are iron, calcium, vitamin D, vitamin B12, zinc, and protein.

Choose a vegetarian eating plan that is low in fat and that provides all of the nutrients your body needs. To replenish food and beverage nutrients that may be lacking in a vegetarian diet some good tips:

Iron: cashews, spinach, lentils, beans, fortified bread or cereal

Calcium: dairy products, fortified soy-based beverages, tofu made with calcium sulphate, collard greens, kale, broccoli

Vitamin D: fortified foods and beverages including milk, soy-based beverages, or cereal

Vitamin B12: eggs, dairy products, fortified cereal or soy-based beverages, tempeh, miso (tempeh/miso are made from soybeans)

Zinc: whole grains (especially the germ and bran of the grain), nuts, tofu, leafy vegetables (spinach, cabbage, lettuce)

Protein: eggs, dairy products, beans, peas, nuts, seeds, tofu, soy-based foods.

One of my particular failings, and the one I have to try hardest with - make sure that you drink plenty of water through the day (but not too much) to keep your body well-hydrated.

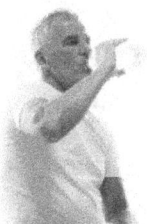

So remember to drink at regular intervals!

1.4 Dairy

Eating Dairy

Regarding dairy products - such as cheeses, yogurts and eggs - for most people these foods can improve bone health and control hypertension. If you are lactose intolerant of course - you will know to avoid these in your diet already.

Dairy products are in general rather fattening and not always healthy. Low-fat and fat-free milk, yogurt, and cheese are just as nutritious as whole-milk dairy products, but they are lower in fat and calories.

Dairy products do have many nutrients your body benefits from - offering protein to build muscles and help organs work properly, and calcium to strengthen bones.

Most milk and some yogurts are now fortified with vitamin D to help your body use the calcium.

Not Eating Dairy

If you cannot digest lactose (the sugar found in dairy products), choose low-lactose or lactose-free dairy products, or other foods and beverages that offer calcium and vitamin D (listed below):

For calcium, use soy-based beverages or tofu made with calcium sulphate, canned salmon, and dark leafy greens, like collards or curly kale.

For vitamin D, use soy-based beverage or cereal (getting sunlight on your skin also gives you a small amount of vitamin D – and it does not have to be a clear sunny day to gain the necessary effect).

Research shows that people who follow a vegetarian eating plan, on average, eat fewer calories and less fat than non-vegetarians. They also tend to have lower body weights relative to their heights than non-vegetarians.

Choosing a vegetarian eating plan with a low fat content may be helpful for weight loss.

1.5 Food To Avoid

There are also certain types of food that we should try to refrain from eating on a regular basis if we want to enjoy good health over 50.

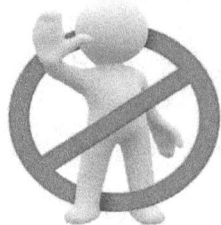

The main group I advise avoiding are processed foods, easy but dangerous. They are generally processed using white sugar, baked goods made from processed flour, foods with high salt content, smoked foods, high-carbohydrate foods, canned foods, canned beverages and processed juices.

One indicator I quite like – '3 ounces of meat or poultry is the size of a deck of cards' (easy to remember that).

As we all know we should not consume alcohol excessively (personally I believe moderation is okay and can even be beneficial), or we should refrain from indulging in any kind of tobacco products of course. Starches are fattening and should be limited when trying to lose weight. Many foods high in starch, like bread, rice, pasta, cereals, beans, fruits, and some vegetables (potatoes, yams) are low in fat and calories.

They become high in fat and calories when eaten in large portion sizes or when covered with high-fat toppings like butter, sour cream, or mayonnaise.

1.6 Diets

I am not a big fan of diets as such, especially ones that strictly limit calories or food choices. Most people quickly get tired of them and regain any lost weight. Fad diets may be unhealthy because they may not provide all of the nutrients your body needs.

Also, losing weight at a very rapid rate (more than 3 pounds a week after the first couple of weeks) may well increase your risk for developing gallstones (clusters of solid material in the gallbladder that can be extremely painful).

Diets that provide less than 800 calories per day also could result in heart rhythm abnormalities.

No foods can burn fat. Some foods with caffeine may speed up your metabolism (the way your body uses energy, or calories) for a short time, but they do not cause weight loss.

The best way to lose weight is to cut back on the number of calories you eat and be more physically active.

A weight-loss product that claims to be "natural" or "herbal" is not necessarily safe. These products are not usually scientifically tested to prove that they are safe or that they work.

Making sensible food choices, eating moderate portions, and building physical activity into your daily life is the best way to lose weight and keep it off.

By adopting healthy eating and physical activity habits, you may also lower your risk for developing type 2 diabetes, heart disease, and high blood pressure.

If you are underweight, you may not be getting enough nutrients. Talk to your doctor about the best way to gain weight naturally and meet your nutritional needs.

Even if you do not need to lose weight, you should still follow healthy eating and physical activity habits to help prevent weight gain and keep you healthy over the coming years.

Eat just enough food to satisfy, not to feel full.

1.7 Get a Food Routine

Something I am still trying to force myself into - I know routine is a word with certain connotations for us 'oldies', but in this case it is good to establish a routine, not too rigid, but as a template for ensuring regular healthy eating.

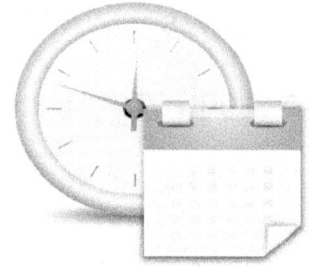

Foods high in starch (also called complex carbohydrates) are an important source of energy for your body.

To help stay on track with a healthy eating plan then, follow my 10 step tips:

1. Don't skip meals. Skipping meals may cause your metabolism to slow down or lead you to eat more high-calorie, high-fat foods at your next meal or snack.

2. Select high-fibre foods like whole-grain breads and cereals, beans, vegetables, and fruits. They should help keep you regular and lower your risk for chronic diseases, such as coronary heart disease and type 2 diabetes.

3. Choose lean beef, turkey breast, fish, or chicken with the skin removed to lower the amount of fat and calories in your meals. As you age, your body needs fewer calories, especially if you are not very active.

4. Have one or two servings of low-fat or fat-free milk, yogurt, or cheese every day. As milk products are high in calcium and vitamin D they help to keep your bones strong as you age. If you have trouble digesting or do not like milk products (ie. lactose intolerant), then try reduced-lactose milk products, or soy-based beverages, or even tofu.

5. Choose foods fortified with vitamin B12. Over the age of 50 we sometimes have difficulty absorbing adequate amounts of this vitamin. Therefore, we should get this nutrient through fortified foods, such as breakfast cereals, or from a dietary supplement.

6. Keep nutrient-rich snacks like dried fruit, whole-wheat crackers, or even peanut butter close at hand. Eat only small amounts of such foods because they are high in calories. Limit how often you have high-fat and high-sugar snacks like cake, candy, chips, and soda (treat these as treats).

7. Drink plenty of water or water-based fluids. You may notice that you feel less thirsty as you get older, but don't be fooled - your body still needs water to stay healthy. Examples of water-based fluids are tea and coffee, soup, and low-fat or skim milk.

8. Cook homemade meals in advance and freeze portions to have healthy and easy meals on hand for days when you do not feel like cooking, or are too busy to spare the time.

9. Keep a supply of fresh or frozen herbs and vegetables, and fruits on hand for quick and healthy additions to meals.

10. Try new recipes using different herbs and spices to spark your interest in new food. And even consider setting the table with a nice cloth and a flower in a vase to make mealtime more special.

Pick up leaflets at your local surgery which related advice.

Chapter 2 – Exercise Your Body

Eating the right food and getting rid of bad habits can help you overcome a lot of health problems, but you still need to lead an active lifestyle to achieve optimal health.

Regular exercise will improve your blood circulation, stimulate the metabolism, tone and strengthen your muscles, and burn excess calories.

Experts recommend at least 150 minutes each week of moderately intense physical activity, so what does this mean, and what is the appropriate exercise for you?

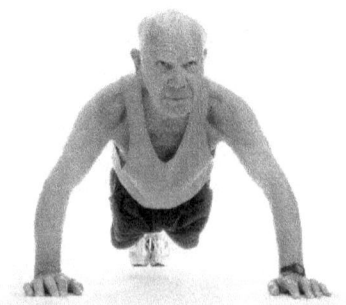

It is recommended that you do around 30 minutes cardiovascular exercises every day.

Try to do at least 30 minutes of moderate-intensity physical activity (like brisk walking) on most days of the week. To lose weight, or to maintain weight loss, you will likely need to do more than 30 minutes of moderate physical activity daily.

Also try to do some strengthening activities two or three times a week. These activities are important because older adults lose muscle and bone every year. Strengthening activities may help prevent or lessen this loss.

Fitting in physical activity to your daily routine is not as hard as you may think, and you do not have to do the whole 30 minutes at one time. Divide those 150 minutes up over the week as your schedule allows.

Remember - it is never too late to start moving about more. Physical activity may help you manage health problems like arthritis, osteoporosis (bone loss), and coronary heart disease. Mobility will help to:

- Keep your body flexible.
- Keep your bones and muscles strong.
- Keep your heart and lungs healthy.

Control high blood sugar, especially if you lose weight.

Let you keep living in your own home without help.

If you have chronic health problems such as coronary heart disease, high blood pressure, diabetes, osteoporosis, or obesity, talk to your GP before starting a vigorous physical activity program, but not really necessary before starting a less strenuous activity like walking.

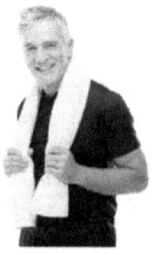

Physical activity can be fun, you just need to figure out which activities you enjoy most. The more enjoyable it is, the more likely you are to stick with it. Some ideas include:

- Walking or taking an exercise class with a friend or in a group – this way, you can cheer each other on, have company, and feel safer when you are outdoors.
- Starting a small garden at home, or in a community allotment.
- Breaking physical activity into short blocks of time - like taking three 10-minute walks during your day - may be easier than taking one 30-minute walk.
- Perform different activities throughout the week to stay interested.

If you are not comfortable being active outdoors because of safety concerns, consider joining your local recreation or fitness center or going to a relative's neighbourhood to walk.

There are lots of ways to be physically active that are free or low-cost:

1. Finding a local park or school track where you can walk.

2. Walking around a mall.

3. Being active with your grandchildren—take a walk, toss a softball, or ride bikes.

4. Walking your dog or meeting up with a neighbour to walk together.

5. Swimming - even if you are not a strong swimmer, join the local club and make a start. And don't be shy - it is never too late to get a swimming lesson, and it is such a great way to take pressure off tired and aching joints (this I know).

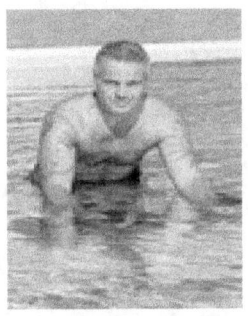

6. If this is all a bit sudden, check out a fitness

video from the library and follow along to the

advice at home, when you are alone.

No matter how busy you are, there are ways to fit in

the 30 minutes or more of physical activity each day.

And try and remember to move around every hour or

so rather than staying in one position for long periods.

Take a break from the computer and make this a

habit.

Set aside some time to be extra active. For instance, if you make it part of your daily routine to walk after breakfast, you will soon not think twice about doing it, and miss it if the severe weather prevents you from venturing outside. Then use the stairs rather than the elevator for at least part of your journey!

Walk to do your errands, whenever possible, leave the car in the driveway.

Be active while doing other things. For example, you can lift weights or march in place while watching TV, or walk around your home while talking on a mobile or cell phone.

Strengthening activities are good for everyone - and there are ways to become stronger without lifting weights. Strength training may help you perform your daily activities with more ease. Consider:

Doing step-ups or wall push-ups in the comfort of your own home.

Using canned foods or filled water bottles as weights.

Walking up and down the stairs - lifting your body weight strengthens your legs and hips.

Physical activity is good for your health at every age. If you have never been active, starting regular physical activity now will improve your strength, endurance, and flexibility.

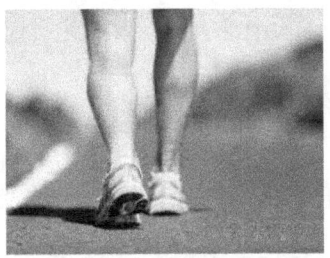

Whatever activity you choose, follow the safety tips below:

Take time to warm up, cool down, and stretch.

Start slowly and build up to more intense activity.

Stop the activity if you experience pain, dizziness, or shortness of breath. Drink plenty of water.

When you are active outdoors, wear lightweight clothes in the summer and layers of clothing in the winter.

Wear sunscreen, sunglasses, and a hat for sun protection.

Wear shoes that fit well and are right for your activity.

Lifting weights or doing strengthening activities like push-ups and crunches on a regular basis will help you maintain or lose weight. These activities will help you build muscle, and muscle burns more calories than body fat.

So if you have more muscle, you burn more calories - even sitting still. Doing strengthening activities 2 or 3 days a week will not "bulk you up." Only intensive strength training, combined with a certain genetic background, can build very large muscles.

If you would prefer (like I do) - carry out household or garden tasks that require you to lift or dig. Strength training helps keep your bones strong while building muscle, which can help burn calories.

It is also advisable to seek a full medical check-up when you reach the age of 50, and request regular screenings every 2-3 years after that.

You know your body better than anyone else. When you visit your health care team always tell them about any seeming insignificant changes in your health, including your vision and hearing.

Ask about checking for any condition you are concerned about, not just the ones we mention here. If you are wondering about diseases such as glaucoma, prostate cancer, or skin cancer, for example, ask about them.

Using aspirin has become a hot topic. Ask your doctor about taking aspirin to prevent heart disease. There has been a lot of recent press about the benefits of aspirin in counteracting certain health conditions, such as heart disease, but as always learn more about this as there are always potential side effects if you take 'chemicals' on a regular basis.

Achieve a healthy weight and stay there. Balance the calories you take in from food and drink with the calories you burn off by your activities.

Be tobacco free. If you smoke it is time to seriously consider the dangers to your health as you get older - talk to someone about how to cut down but ideally quit!

If you drink alcohol, have no more than one or two drinks a day, and have days without, to rest your liver. If you are older than 65, limit this to no more than one drink a day. A standard drink is one 12-ounce bottle of beer or a glass of wine, or a small glass of spirits.

Oh, and remember to get a good night's sleep. Sleep can do a lot of healing to a tired body at the end of a busy day.

Chapter 3 - Weight Balance

What is a healthy weight for men over 50?

There is no right answer of course, but maintaining a healthy weight will reduce the risk of many chronic diseases. It may also help you move better and stay mentally sharp.

If you are underweight, overweight, or obese, you are at risk for certain health problems. Aside from online research, ask your health care provider to determine a healthy weight for you.

If you start to gain or lose weight and do not know why, your health care provider can tell you if this change is healthy for you.

Overweight

If you are overweight or inactive, you may have a higher risk of:

- type 2 diabetes (high blood sugar)

- high blood pressure

- coronary heart disease

- stroke

- osteoarthritis

- certain forms of cancer

- fatty liver disease

- sleep apnea (interrupted breathing during sleep)

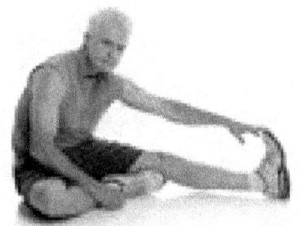

Being physically active and making smart food choices is good for your health. In addition to improving your physical health, moving more and eating better may also give you more energy to live your daily life and:

- Reduce stress.
- Help you feel better about yourself.
- Relieve boredom or depression.
- Set an example for your family, and friends too.

On that last point, your family and friends can be great sources of motivation and support as you adopt a healthier lifestyle.

Ask them to join you in healthy eating and physical activity - it is important for them, too.

By making healthy choices together, it will become easier to eat right and be active.

If you are overweight, losing as little as 5 percent of your body weight will lower your risk for several diseases, including coronary heart disease and type 2 diabetes.

To lose weight and keep it off over time, try to make long-term changes in your eating and physical activity habits, rather than just following a fad diet.

So, if you weigh 200 pounds, this will mean losing 10 pounds. Slow and steady weight loss of 1/2 to 2 pounds per week, and not more than 3 pounds per week, is the safest way to lose weight.

The key to successful weight loss is making changes in your eating and physical activity habits that you can keep up for the rest of your life.

If you do need to lose weight, make sure that you reduce your total calories, but do not reduce your nutrient intake.

But diets that strictly limit calories or food choices are hard to follow, and most people quickly get tired of them and regain any lost weight.

Losing weight at a very rapid rate (more than 3 pounds a week after the first couple of weeks) may increase your risk for developing gallstones (clusters of solid material in the gallbladder that can be extremely painful).

A weight-loss product that claims to be "natural" or "herbal" is not necessarily safe. These products are not usually scientifically tested to prove that they are safe for the average user.

I recommend that you talk with your GP before using any weight-loss product. Some natural or herbal weight-loss products can be harmful.

Research suggests that losing 1/2 to 2 pounds a week by making healthy food choices, eating moderate portions, and building physical activity into your daily life is the best way to lose weight and, critically, to keep it lost.

By adopting healthy eating and physical activity habits, you also lower your risk for developing type 2 diabetes, heart disease, and high blood pressure.

Underweight

There are other health risks from being underweight too, such as:

- decreased immunity
- poor memory
- osteoporosis (bone loss)
- decreased muscle strength
- hypothermia (lowered body temperature)
- even constipation

If you are underweight, you may not be getting enough nutrients. Again, talk to your doctor about the best way to gain weight naturally and meet your nutritional needs.

Even if you do not need to lose weight, you should still follow healthy eating and physical activity habits to help prevent weight gain and keep you healthy over the coming years.

Chapter 4 - Exercise Your Mind

One historically underestimated and less understood health factor in growing older is the area of mental agility and brain health.

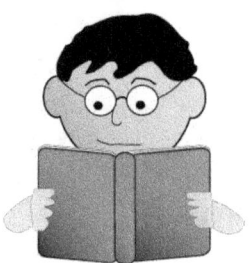

Also, you should engage in some mentally-stimulating activities on a regular basis to keep your mind sharp and healthy.

Mental exercise is always beneficial, but becomes more important for us as we grow older. When we are young we naturally, and largely without knowing it, get plenty of brain exercise in our busy and challenging (yes kids!) daily lives.

As we get older, however, and maybe our daily mental challenges ease off, we should make some conscious attempt to flex the brain muscles on a very regular basis.

This will help to slow down the mental ageing process and is just as important as the physical exercising we talked about above.

Some useful habits that will help to keep our minds alert:

- Crosswords

- Sudoku

- Other mind puzzles (check the newspaper)

- Jigsaw puzzles

- Reading, and writing

- Web browsing

Using the Internet is a great new addition to keeping active at home, interspersed with movement away from the laptop or tablet of course!

Another activity to consider seriously (and I am not biased of course) is writing. Whether it is sending out emails, or writing physical letters to your friends or relatives make the effort today.

Putting your thoughts down on paper can be quite liberating.

Also try to extend your choice of reading materials to include a topic you have always been interested in but never quite got round to - such as history, biography, or cooking..

If you decide to try your hand at more serious writing, join a local writers' club or go on amazon and check out direct publishing (hello - it really is quite straightforward as I know from publishing this book).

There is at least one book in everyone.

Or why not take up an evening class doing something which you would not normally think of doing, or have always wanted to do but never had the time.

Finally, what about having a clear out at home - tidy up all of the things you have managed to collect over the last forty years, relive old memories and celebrate all of your achievements.

Compile the videos, and reorganise your collection of 'stuff'.

Chapter 5 - Common Health Concerns

Here I want to discuss some of the more common concerns and potential afflictions which affect men once they pass the age of 50 (if not before).

1. Depression

Some warning signs:

- Do you feel tired and irritable all the time? Have you lost interest in your work, family, or hobbies, or sex?
- Are you having trouble sleeping and feeling angry or aggressive, or strangely sad? Have you been feeling like this for weeks or months?

If so, then you may have depression.

Everyone feels sad or irritable sometimes, or has trouble sleeping occasionally. But these feelings and troubles usually pass after a couple of days, and best not to worry unduly.

When a man has depression, he has trouble with daily life and loses interest in anything for weeks at a time. Men may suffer depression differently to women, and are more likely to feel very tired and irritable, and lose interest in their work, family, or hobbies. They may be more likely to have difficulty sleeping than women who have depression.

Many men do not recognize, acknowledge, or seek help for their depression. They are certainly more reluctant to talk about how they are feeling. But depression is a real and treatable illness. With the right treatment, most men with depression can get better and gain back their interest in work, family, and hobbies.

Several factors may contribute to depression in men in particular:

- Genes - a family history of depression.
- Brain chemistry – in fact brains of those with depression look visibly different on scans than those of people without the illness.
- Stress - loss of a loved one, a difficult relationship or any stressful situation may trigger depression in some men.

Most of the time, it is probably a combination of all these factors.

The first step to getting the right treatment for depression is to visit a doctor or mental health professional. He or she can do an exam or lab tests to rule out other conditions that may have the same symptoms as depression. The doctor will also tell if certain medications you are taking may be affecting your mood.

For medication, anti-depressants can work well to treat depression. But they may take several weeks to have any positive effect. And they can have side effects including - headaches, nausea, difficulty sleeping, nervousness and agitation. These will lessen over time, but talk to your doctor about any side effects that you may be having.

Some therapies – such as Cognitive Behavioural Therapy (CBT) - are just as effective as medications for certain types of depression. Therapy helps by teaching new ways of thinking and behaving, and changing habits that may be contributing to the depression it can help men to understand and work through difficult situations or relationships that may be causing their depression or making it worse.

If you are unsure where to go for help, again ask your family doctor. You can also check the phone book for mental health professionals or in the US you can check with your insurance carrier to find someone who participates in your plan.

For the latest information on medications, visit the US Food and Drug Administration website (link in References). Not everyone responds to treatment the same way.

Medications may need to be combined with on-going talk therapy, or may need to be changed or adjusted to minimise side effects and achieve the best results. If you think you are depressed or know someone who is, don't lose hope. Seek help for depression (and see the NIMH link below).

2. Strokes and Heart Problems

There is often confusion as to what constitutes a stroke so I will cover it briefly here as it is pertinent. A stroke occurs when the blood supply to part of the brain is suddenly interrupted, such as when a blood vessel bursts or a clot blocks blood flow.

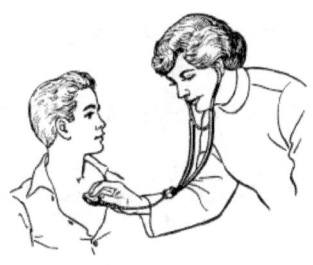

Although strokes occur in and damage the brain, they can affect the whole body. Strokes may cause paralysis (the complete or partial loss of the ability to move), speech problems, or the inability to complete daily tasks. Sometimes these effects are temporary and sometimes they are permanent.

Stroke survivors will need rehabilitation, therapy that helps people relearn skills or learn new skills – recovery success is unique for each person.

Many people require mental health treatment after a stroke to address depression, anxiety, frustration, or anger. Several factors may affect the risk and severity of depression after a stroke, including:

Stroke and heart disease share the same risk factors, such as high blood pressure and being overweight. One recent study showed that older people with heart disease who had more severe and frequent depression symptoms were more likely to have a stroke.

3. Failing Vision

While getting old is unavoidable, sadly, losing your vision doesn't have to be.

One condition - Presbyopia, or "aging vision," as it is commonly referred to - is the hardening of the lens and tightening of the eye muscles associated with aging.

This condition occurs in nearly everyone at some point in their lives, typically around the age of 40. Aging vision causes the ciliary muscle, which is the muscle that is responsible for focusing, to become inflexible. It is therefore unable to change the shape of the lens the amount required to focus on near-point objects. At first you might find it hard to focus on the newspaper or on a menu (sound familiar?) at a restaurant. Before you know it, your arms aren't long enough to read anything.

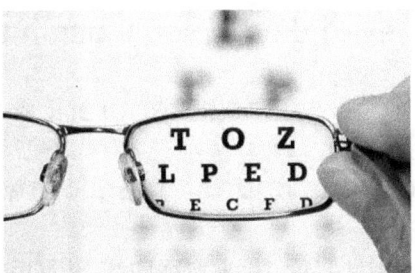

You might then decide to go and get your first pair of reading glasses - your optician or local drugstore is happy as you have just become a lifelong customer!

If you suffer from presbyopia, you can manage it.

What do you do when you have a tight hamstring or bicep? You stretch it out every day, and over time, it regains its flexibility and elasticity. Well, your eyes are no different.

There are special optical exercises and vision-improvement techniques (eg Vision Therapy) that can help you regain the elasticity that your eyes once had and the clear, natural vision that you remember from years ago.

And when you do the exercises, in just a few weeks (sometimes even days), you'll begin to stop the vicious cycle of eyesight deterioration and start to notice tremendous improvements in your vision.

Imagine enjoying the newspaper without searching the house for your glasses. Or celebrating at a special restaurant without having to hold the menu at arm's length!

4. Hearing Loss

Probably not going to affect you just yet, but it is worth a mention, especially as men are more likely to experience hearing loss than women.

Hearing loss is a common problem caused by noise, aging, disease, and heredity. Hearing is a complex sense involving both the ear's ability to detect sounds and the brain's ability to interpret those sounds, including the sounds of speech.

Some factors that may determine how much hearing loss will negatively affect a person's quality of life are the history of exposures to loud noise, and environmental or drug-related toxins that are harmful to hearing.

Hearing loss is one of the most common conditions affecting older adults - about 30 million American adults report some degree of hearing loss.

There is a strong relationship between aging and reported hearing loss: 18% of American adults 45-64 years old, 30% of adults 65-74 years old, and 47% of adults 75 years old, or older, have a hearing impairment.

People with hearing loss may find it hard to have a conversation with friends and family, or respond to alarm noises.

Hearing loss comes in many forms. It can range from a mild loss in which a person misses certain high-pitched sounds, such as the voices of women and children, to a total loss of hearing. It can be hereditary or it can result from disease, trauma, certain medications, or long-term exposure to loud noises.

There are two general categories of hearing loss: Sensorineural hearing loss occurs when there is damage to the inner ear or the auditory nerve. This type of hearing loss is usually permanent.

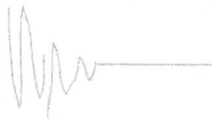

Conductive hearing loss occurs when sound waves cannot reach the inner ear. The cause may commonly be caused by an earwax build-up, fluid, or a punctured eardrum. Medical treatment or surgery can usually restore conductive hearing loss

Tinnitus, common in older people, is a ringing, roaring, clicking, hissing, or buzzing sound. It can come and go. It might be heard in one or both ears and be loud or soft.

But tinnitus is a symptom, not a disease. It can accompany any type of hearing loss. It can be a side effect of medications. Something as simple as a piece of earwax blocking the ear canal can cause tinnitus, but it can also be the result of a number of health conditions.

If you think you have tinnitus, see your doctor. You may be referred to an otolaryngologist - a surgeon who specializes in ear, nose, and throat diseases - (commonly called an ear, nose, and throat doctor, or an ENT). The ENT will physically examine your head, neck, and ears and test your hearing to determine the appropriate treatment.

Hearing loss left unattended can lead to other problems, so try not to be one of those guys who do not want to admit they have trouble hearing.

If you can't hear well you may become depressed or may withdraw from others to avoid feeling frustrated or embarrassed about not understanding what is being said. So get it checked out.

Sometimes older people are mistakenly thought to be confused, unresponsive, or uncooperative just because they don't hear well.

Hearing problems that are ignored or untreated can get worse. If you have a hearing problem, you can get help. See your doctor. Hearing aids, special training, certain medicines, and surgery are some of the choices that can help people with hearing problems.

5. Other Aging 'Shadows'

I call them the aging 'shadows' as they are 2 man problems (well apart from impotency which I won't cover as it is widely covered elsewhere) things we all become conscious of as we get older.

I will briefly talk about the 2 types of cancer in older men:

Bowel cancer

If you've had blood in your stools or looser pooh for 2-3 weeks, your doctor should be consulted. Chances are it's nothing to worry about, but these symptoms could be signs of bowel cancer, so do tell your doctor. As with other ailments, finding bowel cancer early makes it more treatable and could save your life.

Bowel cancer is the UK's second most common cancer, with around 30,000 new cases each year. Bowel cancer affects both men and women, and nine out of ten people diagnosed with the disease are over 50. Those with a family history of bowel cancer are more at risk. Other bowel cancer symptoms include:

A pain or lump in your tummy

Feeling more tired than usual for some time

Losing weight for no obvious reason

Being a man will often mean that we delay getting health issues checked out. Remember, you are not wasting anyone's time by getting your symptoms checked out and, if it's not serious, your mind will be put at rest.

However, if it turns out to be a condition such as bowel cancer, early detection can make all the difference. Over 90% of those diagnosed with early stage bowel cancer are successfully treated. A trip to your doctor's surgery could save your life.

Prostate cancer

The prostate is a doughnut shaped gland located in the male pelvis, at the base of the bladder. We all have them, but will only really notice it when it goes wrong! It grows as we do, and will be about 50g by the time we reach 50.

Its main function is to make some of the nutritional fluid of semen - about 30% of the total fluid which accompanies sperm in ejaculation. Without prostate fluid those sperms would not travel very far.

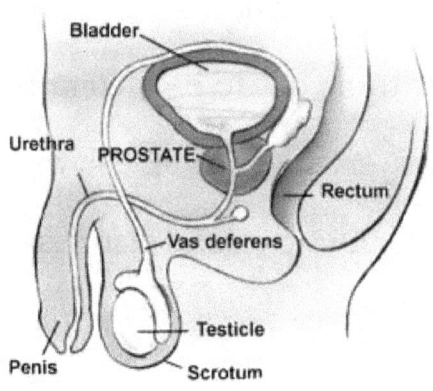

There are three main things that could go wrong with your prostate:

1. enlargement – "Benign Prostatic Hyperplasia" or "BPH" is the technical term.

2. cancer growth.

3. inflammation - known as "prostatitis".

With any prostate problem, it is important you talk to your doctor to see what your symptoms mean. GPs have been provided with a resource pack to talk to you if you are worried about prostate cancer.

The risk of prostate cancer gets higher in older men. Symptoms are similar to other prostate problems, particularly difficulty in passing urine, but other symptoms include lower back pain, pain in the hips or pelvis, erection problems and, more rarely, blood in the urine.

All these symptoms can also be caused by other problems. Prostate cancer behaves differently in different men, with some growing very slowly and some growing quickly. As of yet - there are no known measures you can take to reduce your risk of prostate cancer, but the important thing is to catch it early.

Summary

Healthy eating, regular physical activity and mental exercises are the keys to good health at any age. They will lower the risks of obesity, type 2 diabetes, coronary heart disease, cancer, and other chronic diseases. They may even help ward off depression and will keep your mind sharp as you age.

Consider your current situation and be completely honest with yourself - you may be blissfully unaware that you are eating too much fat and/or cholesterol, which can raise heart disease risk.

You may not be eating enough variety and too little fruits vegetables, and whole grains, which may lead to bowel problems due to lack of dietary fibre.

A reduced-calorie eating plan that includes recommended amounts of carbohydrate, protein, and fat may also allow you to lose weight, but that is for more serious consideration.

And do not be afraid to talk to your doctor or GP for more specific advice if you have particular health problems or concerns.

Remember, it is never too late to make healthy changes in your life.

Just Get Started Today!

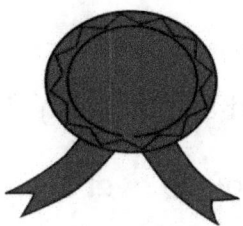

By following a healthy and balanced eating plan, you will not have to stop eating whole classes of foods, and miss out on some key nutrients they contain. You will also find it easier to stick with an eating plan that includes a greater variety of foods.

In summary then - a healthy eating plan is one that:

Emphasizes fruits, vegetables, whole grains, and fat-free or low-fat milk and milk products.

Includes a variety of lean meats, poultry, fish, beans, eggs, and nuts.

Is low in saturated fats, trans fat, cholesterol, salt (sodium), and added sugars.

Is varied and interesting enough to keep you satisfied.

Eating the right food and getting rid of bad habits will definitely help you to overcome a lot of health problems.

You still need to lead an active lifestyle to achieve optimal health. Regular exercise can improve your blood circulation, stimulate metabolism, tone and strengthen your muscles, and burn excess calories.

Become and remain tobacco free - if you do still smoke it is never too late to consider further reducing your habit - talk to someone about how to cut down but ideally quit!

If you drink alcohol, as indeed I do, have no more than one or two drinks a day, and ensure you have at least 2 days a week of abstinence to rest your liver. Oh, and remember to get a good night's sleep. Sleep can do a lot of healing to a tired body at the end of a busy day.

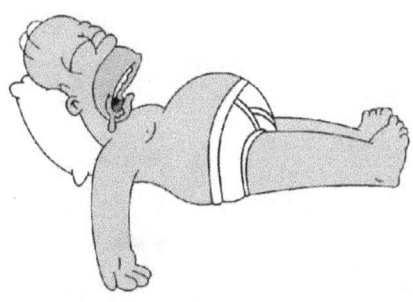

Appendix 1 - Get Walking

Walking is one of the easiest and rewarding ways for you to be physically active. It is inexpensive and you can walk almost anywhere and at any time, yes, in any weather as long as you are prepared.

Here are some general tips on how to create and follow a walking plan. Even if you do no other conscious exercise, walking will give you more energy and stamina and crucially will lift your mood, tone your muscles and strengthen your bones.

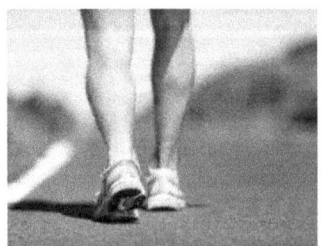

It will also help to increase the number of calories your body uses.

Prepare for walking by asking yourself -

Has your health care provider told you that you have heart trouble, diabetes, or asthma?

When you are physically active, do you have pains in your chest, neck, shoulder, or arm?

Do you often feel faint or have dizzy spells?

Do you feel extremely breathless after you have been physically active?

Has your health care provider told you that you have bone or joint problems, such as arthritis?

Are you over 50 years old and not used to doing any moderate physical activity?

Do you smoke?

Do you have a health problem or physical reason not mentioned here that might keep you from starting a regular walking program?

If you answered "yes" to any of these questions, check with your health care provider before starting a walking program.

Leave time in your schedule to follow a walking program that will work for you:

Choose a safe place to walk.

Wear shoes with proper arch support, a firm heel, and thick flexible soles.

They will cushion your feet and absorb shock.

Wear clothes that will keep you dry and comfortable.

Put on fabrics that absorb sweat and therefore remove it from your skin.

Divide your walk into three parts. Warm up slowly, then increase your speed to a brisk walk. This means walking fast enough to elevate your heart rate while still being able to speak comfortably, concentrate, and breathe without effort.

Cool down slowly.

Stretch lightly after warm-up and cool-down.

Spread your walking evenly throughout the week. Try to walk at least 3 days each week if you cannot walk daily. Each week, add a few minutes to your walk. Break up your walk into multiple sessions throughout the day if you have a busy schedule.

Make sure each session is at least 10 minutes long. To avoid stiff or sore muscles and joints, start gradually. Over several weeks, begin walking faster, going further, and taking longer walks.

Consider keeping track of your progress with a walking journal or log.

Record the date, time, and of course the distance. Experts recommend at least 150 minutes each week of moderately intense physical activity.

Divide these minutes up over the week as your schedule allows. Review the guide on the back of this brochure for suggestions on beginning and gradually building your walking program.

Keep safety in mind as you plan when and where you walk. If you walk at dawn, dusk, or night, wear a reflective vest or brightly coloured clothing.

Walk in a group when possible and carry some identification with you, as well as a way to contact someone if you need help.

Notify family and friends of your group's walking time and route. Do not wear jewellery or headphones.

Be aware of your surroundings.

Walking with proper form is very important, walk with your chin up and your shoulders slightly back.

Let the heel of your foot touch the ground first, then roll your weight forward.

Walk with your toes pointed forward.

Swing your arms naturally as you walk.

Take a daily walk, however short it may be.

If you are walking fewer than three times per week, give yourself more than two weeks before increasing the pace and frequency.

Stretch gently after you warm up your muscles, and again after you cool down. Stretching exercises (see below) can increase your range of motion and allow you to do more of the things you need to do.

Stretching by itself is not designed to enhance strength or endurance, however keeping one's muscles more flexible can also reduce strains which could help prevent injuries and falling, and should improve circulation as well.

Appendix 2 - Start Stretching

Try doing these 4 simple stretches. Do not hold your

breath when you stretch, perform slow movements

and stretch only as far as you feel comfortable.

Side Reach:

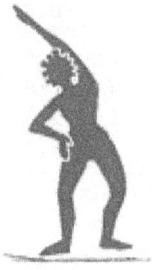

Reach one arm over your head and over to the side.

Keep your hips steady and your shoulders

straight to the side.

Hold for 10 seconds and repeat on the other side.

Wall Push:

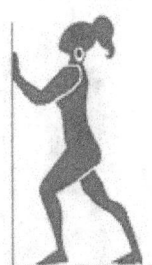

Lean your hands on a wall and place your feet about 3

to 4 feet away from the wall. Bend one knee and point

it towards the wall.

Keep your back leg straight with your foot flat and

your toes pointed straight ahead.

Hold for 10 seconds and repeat with the other leg.

Knee Pull:

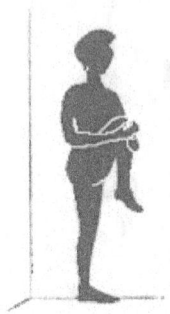

Lean your back against a wall.

Keep your head, hips, and feet in a straight line.

Pull one knee toward your chest, hold for 10 seconds,

and then repeat with the other leg.

Hamstring Stretch:

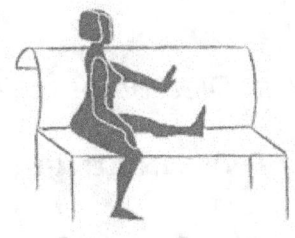

Sit on a garden bench or hard surface so that one leg

is stretched out on the bench with your toes pointing

up. Keep your other foot flat on the ground.

Straighten your back, and if you feel a stretch in the

back of your thigh, hold for 10 seconds and then

change sides and repeat.

If you do not feel a stretch, slowly lean forward from

your hips until you feel a stretch.

Useful References

American Dietetic Association

http://www.eatright.org

Food and Nutrition Information - USDA

http://www.nal.usda.gov/fnic

Fit and Fabulous as You Mature

http://www.win.niddk.nih.gov/publications/ma

ture.htm

Weight Loss for Life

http://www.win.niddk.nih.gov/publications/for

_life.htm

Guides for healthy living, encyclopaedia of health-

related topics, health news.

http://healthfinder.gov

Healthy Men. An AHRQ Web site for men on staying

healthy.

http://www.ahrq.gov/healthymen

About the Author

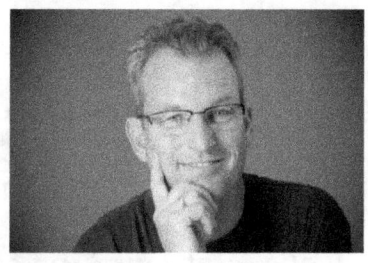

CW Piper is a man of varying talents, and has worked in a wide (very wide) spectrum of jobs throughout his career, from kitchen porter to bar manager, journalist to writer, Ireland to Australia, and back again. He is for now settled with 2 grown up children living in Buckinghamshire, England.

He has many interests, from finance to music, travel to cooking, tragedy to comedy, and always tries hard to see the funny side of life.

*'If you liked my book and have a minute - I'd really appreciate a **review.***

This is the first in a series on health related issues.

*To follow my antics and heed my eternally optimistic advice.. visit my website at **cwpiper.com**, or do find me and chat friend up on **facebook**.*